THE ULTIMATE GRILL DIET COOKBOOK

Transforming Your Health, One Flame at a Time

Adams .U. Morris

TABLE OF CONTE NTS

Chapter 1...5

Introduction to Grill Diets 5

Chapter 2...15

Types of Grills...................................15

Chapter 3...28

Essential Grilling Equipment 28

Chapter 4...42

Grilling Techniques......................42

Chapter 5...59

Grilling Recipes - Meat 59

Chapter 6...77

Grilling Recipes - Seafood and Vegetables.............................77

Chapter 7.............................94

Grilling Sauces, Marinades, and Rubs 94

Chapter 8.............................110

Grill Diet - Tips for Success.........110

Conclusion 126

CHAPTER 1

Introduction to Grill Diets

Grilling is more than just a way of cooking food; it's a culinary tradition deeply embedded in cultures around the world. It's a method that combines flavor, simplicity, and a connection to nature that few other cooking techniques can match. In this first chapter, we embark on a journey into the heart of grill diets, exploring what they are, their historical and cultural significance, and how they can serve as a gateway to a healthier lifestyle.

The Essence of a Grill Diet

At its core, a grill diet centers around cooking food over an open flame or on a hot surface, often using a grill. This method imparts a unique smoky flavor and appealing char marks to various foods, from meats and vegetables to seafood and even fruits. Grill diets are not just about the taste, though; they're about embracing a way of cooking that can be both delicious and health-conscious.

The Grilling Tradition: A Historical Perspective

To truly appreciate the grill diet, we must delve into its rich history. Grilling as a cooking technique dates back thousands of years, with evidence of its existence found in ancient civilizations. For instance, the Egyptians grilled meats over open fires, and the Greeks had a fascination with spits and skewers.

However, it's in the Americas where grilling truly took root. Native Americans practiced grilling long before the arrival of European settlers. They would cook everything from game meats to corn over open flames. When European colonists encountered this technique, they adopted it enthusiastically, and the tradition of American barbecues was born.

Cultural Significance of Grilling

Grilling isn't just about the food; it's also a celebration of community and culture. In many parts of the world, grilling is a social event, bringing friends and families together. Think of the summer barbecues in the United States, the Brazilian churrasco, or the South African braai. These gatherings are about more than just cooking; they're a time for bonding and storytelling.

Moreover, grilling often represents a connection to the land and its resources. It's a way of celebrating the harvest and the bounty of nature. In many cultures, grilling has a spiritual dimension, symbolizing the importance of fire and its transformative power in cooking.

Grill Diets: The Path to a Healthier Lifestyle

Now that we've established the cultural and historical roots of grilling, it's time to explore why a grill diet can be a stepping stone to a healthier lifestyle. There are several key reasons for this:

1. **Less Fat, More Flavor**: Grilling allows fat to drip away from the food as it cooks. This means you can enjoy the taste of marbled meats without consuming excessive fats. The result is a flavorful, leaner meal.

2. **Preservation of Nutrients**: Grilling is a quick cooking method that helps preserve the natural nutrients in food. Compared

to boiling or frying, where nutrients can leach into the cooking liquid or oil, grilling retains more of the food's goodness.

3. **Minimal Added Fats**: When marinating or seasoning food for grilling, you can use healthier ingredients like olive oil, herbs, and spices instead of heavy sauces and excessive fats. This reduces the overall calorie count.

4. **Versatile and Balanced**: A grill diet can be incredibly diverse. You can grill a wide range of foods, including

lean proteins like chicken breast, fish, and plant-based options like tofu and vegetables. This variety allows you to maintain a balanced diet.

5. **Portion Control**: Grilling encourages portion control naturally. The time and effort it takes to grill each item make you more mindful of your meal size.

6. **Engaging Outdoor Activity**: Grilling often takes place outdoors, which encourages physical activity and a break from the sedentary indoor lifestyle.

7. **Social and Emotional Well-being**: As mentioned earlier, grilling is often a communal activity. Socializing and enjoying a meal together can contribute to overall well-being and reduced stress.

By embracing a grill diet, you're not just changing the way you cook; you're adopting a holistic approach to food and lifestyle. It's about savoring the flavors of tradition while making conscious choices for your health.

In this chapter, we've scratched the surface of what a grill diet entails. We've discovered its historical roots, cultural significance, and the potential it holds for healthier living. As we progress through this book, we'll delve deeper into the practical aspects of grilling, from the types of grills and essential equipment to mastering grilling techniques and tantalizing recipes that will make your taste buds dance. So, let's fire up those grills and embark on this delicious journey towards a healthier, more flavorful life.

CHAPTER 2

Types of Grills

In the world of grilling, the choice of grill can significantly impact your cooking experience and the flavors you achieve. Chapter 2 of our exploration into grill diets is all about understanding the various types of grills available. From the classic charcoal grill to the convenience of gas and the versatility of electric grills, we'll take a deep dive into the world of grilling equipment.

The Charcoal Grill: A Timeless Classic

Let's start with the most iconic and perhaps the oldest type of grill – the charcoal grill. This classic grill has been a staple in backyards, parks, and campgrounds for generations. The allure of the charcoal grill lies in the primal satisfaction of starting a fire and cooking over glowing embers. Here are some key points to consider:

- **Flavor:** Charcoal grills are revered for imparting a distinct smoky flavor to your food. The charcoal itself can be infused with unique aromas, which are then transferred to your meat, vegetables, or other grillables.

- **Versatility**: Charcoal grills come in various sizes and shapes, from small portable models to large, stationary ones. This versatility allows you to choose the right grill for your cooking needs.

- **Temperature Control**: While they can be a bit more challenging to control compared to gas grills, experienced grillers can manipulate the heat by adjusting the airflow through vents and the arrangement of coals.

- **Authentic Experience**: Many grill enthusiasts appreciate the hands on experience of lighting and tending to charcoal grills. It's a process that connects you with the history and tradition of grilling.

However, it's important to note that charcoal grilling can be time-consuming. It takes some practice to achieve consistent results, and cleanup can be messy. But for those who savor the process as much as the end product, a charcoal grill is often the top choice.

The Gas Grill: Convenience and Precision

Gas grills have gained immense popularity for their ease of use and precision in controlling cooking temperatures. They're often the go-to choice for those seeking convenience without sacrificing flavor. Here's why gas grills are a favorite:

- **Instant Heat**: Gas grills are known for their rapid heating. With the push of a button, you can have your grill ready for cooking within minutes.

- **Temperature Control**: Gas grills offer precise temperature control through adjustable burners. This makes them ideal for cooking a wide range of foods, from delicate fish to hearty steaks.

- **Clean Burning**: Propane or natural gas used in these grills burns cleanly, without producing the smoke and ash associated with charcoal. This means less mess and easier cleanup.

- **Versatility**: Many gas grills come equipped with side burners, rotisserie kits, and additional features, allowing you to expand your grilling repertoire.

While gas grills excel in convenience, some purists argue that they lack the smoky flavor of charcoal grills. However, you can enhance the smokiness by using wood chips or chunks in a smoker box or on the grill grates.

The Electric Grill: Indoor and Compact Outdoor Cooking

Electric grills offer a unique grilling experience, and they are particularly suitable for those living in apartments or areas with strict fire regulations. Here are the key aspects of electric grills:

- **Indoor and Outdoor Use**: Electric grills are versatile in that they can be used indoors, on balconies, or in small outdoor spaces where open flames may not be allowed.

- **Ease of Use**: They are incredibly easy to operate, often requiring only a power outlet. Just plug it in, set the temperature, and you're ready to grill.

- **Smokeless**: Electric grills produce minimal smoke, making them ideal for indoor grilling without setting off smoke alarms.

- **Compact and Portable**: Electric grills come in various sizes, some of which are highly portable, making them suitable for picnics or camping.

However, electric grills may not deliver the same intense sear or smoky flavor as charcoal or gas grills. They are often seen as a

compromise between convenience
and the traditional grilling
experience.

Additional Grill Types and Considerations

Apart from the main three types
mentioned above, there are other
specialized grills to consider:

- **Pellet Grills**: These grills
  use wood pellets as fuel,
  combining the convenience
  of gas with the smoky flavor
  of wood. They offer precise
  temperature control and are
  becoming increasingly
  popular.

- **Kamado Grills**: Inspired by traditional Japanese cooking, Kamado grills are egg-shaped ceramic cookers that excel in both grilling and smoking. They are known for excellent heat retention and versatility.

- **Infrared Grills**: Infrared grills use radiant heat to cook food directly, resulting in even cooking and searing. They are prized for their ability to lock in juices and create impressive grill marks.

- **Hybrid Grills**: Some grills combine multiple fuel

sources, such as charcoal and gas, offering flexibility and flavor options in one unit.

When choosing a grill, it's essential to consider your lifestyle, cooking preferences, available space, and budget. Each type has its advantages, and the "best" grill for you will depend on your individual needs and priorities.

In this chapter, we've covered the main types of grills you'll encounter in your grilling journey. The choice between charcoal, gas, electric, or specialized grills is a significant decision that will influence your cooking style and the flavors you can achieve. As we continue through this book, we'll delve deeper into the specifics of using each type of grill, including essential equipment and techniques to master the art of grilling. So, whether you're drawn to the classic allure of charcoal, the convenience of gas, or the versatility of electric, there's a grill out there waiting to help you savor the flavors of the grill diet.

CHAPTER 3

Essential Grilling Equipment

In Chapter 3 of our journey into the world of grill diets, we shift our focus to the essential equipment and tools that every aspiring grill master should have. While the type of grill you choose is crucial, having the right accessories and equipment can make all the difference in your grilling experience. Let's explore the must-have items for successful grilling:

1. Grilling Utensils: The Basics

First and foremost, you'll need a set of grilling utensils to handle food on the grill and ensure safety. This includes:

- **Tongs**: Long-handled tongs are essential for flipping meats and vegetables on the grill without getting too close to the heat. Look for tongs with a good grip and sturdy construction.
- **Spatula**: A wide spatula with a thin edge is perfect for flipping burgers, fish fillets, or delicate items like grilled

pizza. It helps prevent sticking and tearing.

- **Grill Brush**: Keeping your grill grates clean is vital for flavor and hygiene. A grill brush with stiff bristles will help you remove residue and charred bits.

- **Basting Brush**: If you plan on basting your food with sauces or marinades, a basting brush is indispensable. Look for one with heat-resistant bristles.

- **Grill Fork**: While not as essential as tongs and a spatula, a grill fork can be handy for checking the doneness of meat or moving food around the grill.

2. Thermometers for Precision Cooking

To ensure that your grilled food is cooked to perfection and safe to eat, having a good thermometer is crucial. Here are two types you should consider:

- **Instant-Read Thermometer**: This handheld device provides a quick and accurate temperature reading, allowing you to check the doneness of your food instantly. It's ideal for checking steaks, chicken, or fish.

- **Probe Thermometer**: A probe thermometer has a long, heat-resistant cable with a probe that can be inserted into the meat or food on the grill. The display unit stays outside the grill and provides real-time temperature monitoring. It's perfect for monitoring larger cuts of meat or smoking sessions.

Properly cooked food not only ensures safety but also enhances the flavors of your grill creations.

3. Grill Gloves and Mitts: Safety First

Grilling involves working with high heat, so safety should always be a priority. A pair of heat-resistant grill gloves or mitts will protect your hands and arms from burns. Look for ones that can withstand high temperatures and have a good grip to handle hot grill grates or utensils.

4. Chimney Starter or Electric Starter

If you're using a charcoal grill, a chimney starter or an electric starter is a game-changer. These devices make lighting charcoal quick and effortless. With a chimney starter, you fill it with charcoal, place newspaper or fire starter cubes underneath, and light it. In a short time, your charcoal will be glowing and ready for the grill, without the need for lighter fluid, which can impart undesirable flavors.

5. Grill Cover: Protect Your Investment

If you're leaving your grill outdoors, investing in a grill cover is a wise choice. A grill cover shields your grill from the elements, preventing rust and extending its lifespan. Make sure to choose a cover that's the right size for your grill model.

6. Grill Grates and Cooking Surfaces

While your grill likely comes with its own grates, you can enhance your grilling experience by investing in additional cooking surfaces:

- **Cast Iron Grates**: These provide excellent heat retention and can create beautiful grill marks on your food. They require seasoning and proper care to prevent rust.

- **Grill Griddles**: Perfect for cooking delicate items like seafood or vegetables that might otherwise fall through the grates. They also work well for breakfast items like pancakes and eggs.

- **Pizza Stones**: If you're a fan of grilled pizza, a pizza stone can help you achieve that crispy, wood-fired crust.

7. Smoking Accessories

If you're interested in exploring the world of smoked meats and flavors, consider adding smoking accessories to your arsenal:

- **Wood Chips or Chunks**: Different types of wood chips or chunks, such as hickory, mesquite, or applewood, can impart unique smoky flavors to your food.

- **Smoker Box**: This small box holds the wood chips and is placed on the grill grates. It smolders and releases smoke, infusing your food with a smoky aroma.

8. Drip Pans and Grill Baskets

Drip pans are essential for capturing drippings from meats or vegetables. They prevent flare-ups and help keep your grill clean. Grill baskets are handy for grilling small or delicate items like shrimp, diced vegetables, or even stir-fry.

9. Long-Handled Grill Brush

Maintaining a clean grill is not only crucial for flavor but also for safety. A long-handled grill brush with sturdy bristles will help you remove residue and charred bits from your grates, ensuring even cooking and reducing the risk of flare-ups.

10. Grill Lights

Grilling at night or in low-light conditions can be challenging. Grill lights, which attach to your grill's handle or surface, provide illumination to help you monitor your food's progress and ensure it's cooked to perfection.

11. Meat Injector

If you're passionate about infusing your meats with flavors, a meat injector can be a valuable tool. It allows you to inject marinades, brines, or seasonings directly into the meat, enhancing its taste and juiciness.

12. Grill Table or Workstation

Having a designated area for food prep and plating can make your grilling sessions more organized and enjoyable. Consider a portable grill table or workstation with storage space for your grilling essentials.

In this chapter, we've covered the essential equipment and tools you'll need to embark on your grill diet journey. Whether you're a beginner or an experienced griller, having the right utensils, thermometers, safety gear, and grilling accessories can elevate your skills and help you achieve the best results. Armed with this knowledge and the right equipment, you're ready to move forward in your grilling adventure, exploring various techniques and recipes that will delight your taste buds and those of your family and friends.

CHAPTER 4

Grilling Techniques

In Chapter 4 of our exploration into grill diets, we dive deep into the heart of grilling by delving into essential grilling techniques. Mastering these techniques is key to achieving the perfect sear, flavor infusion, and overall culinary excellence on the grill. Whether you're a novice or a seasoned griller, this chapter will provide valuable insights into the art of grilling.

1. Direct vs. Indirect Grilling

One of the fundamental techniques in grilling is understanding the difference between direct and indirect grilling:

- **Direct Grilling**: In this method, food is placed directly over the heat source, usually high heat. It's ideal for cooking thinner cuts of meat, such as steaks, burgers, and chops, as well as vegetables and smaller items. Direct grilling sears the exterior of the food, creating those coveted grill marks and locking in juices.

- **Indirect Grilling**: Indirect grilling involves cooking food adjacent to the heat source rather than directly over it. This method is perfect for larger cuts of meat like whole chickens, roasts, and racks of ribs. It allows for slow, even cooking without the risk of burning the exterior.

The key to successful grilling is knowing when to use each method. For example, you might start with direct grilling to sear a steak and then finish it indirectly to ensure it's cooked to the desired internal temperature.

2. Smoking and Slow Cooking

Smoking is a technique that adds layers of flavor to your food through the use of wood smoke. Here are the basics:

- **Wood Chips or Chunks**: As mentioned in Chapter 3, different types of wood chips or chunks (hickory, mesquite, cherry, etc.) impart distinct flavors. Soak them in water before using to create smoke.

- **Smoker Box or Foil Pack**: Place the soaked wood chips or chunks in a smoker box or create a foil pack with punctured holes. These go directly on the grill grates, and as they smolder, they release flavorful smoke.

- **Low and Slow**: Smoking requires low, consistent heat. Maintain a temperature between 225°F and 275°F (107°C to 135°C) for longer cooking times, such as when smoking a brisket or ribs.

- **Patience**: Smoking can take several hours, so patience is key. The slow cooking process allows the smoke to penetrate the meat and infuse it with a rich, smoky flavor.

3. Searing for Flavor

Searing is a technique used to lock in juices and create a flavorful crust on the exterior of your meat. Here's how to do it effectively:

- **Preheat the Grill**: Make sure your grill grates are scorching hot before placing the meat on them. This initial burst of high heat is what creates the sear.

- **Oil the Meat, Not the Grates**: Lightly oil your meat with a high-smoke-point oil (like vegetable or canola oil) before placing it on the grill. This helps prevent sticking and promotes even searing.

- **Don't Overcrowd**: Leave space between your items on the grill to ensure proper searing. Crowded grilling can lead to steaming instead of searing.

- **Minimal Flipping**: Resist the urge to flip your meat too frequently. Allow it to sear undisturbed for a few minutes on each side before flipping.

- **Use the Grill Lid**: When searing thicker cuts of meat, like a steak or pork chop, using the grill lid can help trap heat and create a crust.

4. Marinating and Seasoning

Marinating and seasoning your food is essential for enhancing flavor. Here are some tips:

- **Marinating**: Marinades typically consist of oil, acid (like vinegar or citrus juice), and flavorings (herbs, spices, and aromatics). Marinade times can vary, but avoid marinating for too long with highly acidic marinades, as it can break down the meat's texture.

- **Dry Rubs**: Dry rubs are a mix of spices and herbs that are applied directly to the meat's surface. They can add a burst of flavor and create a tasty crust when grilled.

- **Salt**: Don't forget to season your food with salt. Salt not only enhances flavor but also helps tenderize meats by drawing out moisture, which is then reabsorbed, carrying

the seasoning deep into the
meat.

5. Managing Flare-Ups

Flare-ups can occur when fat or
marinades drip onto the grill's
flames, resulting in a sudden burst
of fire. To manage flare-ups:

- **Keep a Spray Bottle of Water Handy**: A spray bottle filled with water can help tame minor flare-ups by quickly dousing the flames. Ensure it's within reach while grilling.
- **Move Food to a Cooler Spot**: If a flare-up persists,

move the food to a cooler part of the grill until the flames subside. Then, return it to the original grilling area.

- **Trim Excess Fat:** Trimming excess fat from meat can reduce the likelihood of flare-ups. Less fat dripping onto the flames means fewer flare-ups to contend with.

6. Resting Your Grilled Food

Resting your grilled food is a critical yet often overlooked step. After removing your food from the grill, let it rest for a few minutes before serving. This allows the juices to redistribute throughout the meat, resulting in juicier, more tender results.

7. Grilling Vegetables and Fruits

Grilling isn't just for meats; it's also an excellent way to enhance the flavors and textures of vegetables and fruits. Here's how to do it:

- **Prep and Season**: Clean and prepare your vegetables and fruits by brushing them with oil and seasoning with salt and pepper or your choice of herbs and spices.

- **Use a Grill Basket**: For smaller or more delicate items like asparagus or sliced bell peppers, consider using a grill basket to prevent them from falling through the grates.

- **Grill Marks**: To achieve those beautiful grill marks, lay the vegetables or fruits diagonally across the grates and avoid overcrowding.

- **Direct or Indirect**: Depending on the item, you can use both direct and indirect grilling methods.

For example, sear vegetables directly over high heat and then move them to a cooler area to finish cooking.

8. The Two-Zone Fire

A technique often used by experienced grillers, the two-zone fire involves creating two distinct temperature zones on your grill:

- **Direct Zone**: One side of the grill is set up for high heat, ideal for searing and quickly cooking items.
- **Indirect Zone**: The other side of the grill is left without direct heat,

providing a cooler area for slow cooking or finishing items that have been seared.

This technique allows for more precise control over cooking and is especially useful when grilling items with varying thicknesses or when you want to keep some food warm while finishing others.

9. Experiment and Adapt

Ultimately, grilling is an art as much as it is a science. While these techniques serve as a foundation, don't be afraid to experiment, adapt, and develop your unique grilling style. Each grill, type of food, and personal preference can influence your approach to grilling.

In this chapter, we've explored essential grilling techniques that will elevate your grill diet experience. From understanding direct and indirect grilling to perfecting the art of searing, smoking, and seasoning, these techniques are the building blocks of becoming a skilled grill master. As you continue your journey into the world of grilling, keep these techniques in mind and let your creativity flourish as you craft delicious and memorable meals on the grill.

CHAPTER 5

Grilling Recipes - Meat

In Chapter 5 of our exploration into grill diets, we delve into the world of grilling recipes, focusing on meats. Grilling meats is a beloved tradition around the world, and it's where the magic of the grill truly comes alive. From perfectly seared steaks to succulent grilled chicken and tender pork, this chapter will guide you through delicious and diverse meat-based recipes to elevate your grill diet.

1. Grilled Steak: Mastering the Basics

Grilling a steak to perfection is a rite of passage for any grill enthusiast. Here's a simple recipe to get you started:

Ingredients:

- Steak of your choice (ribeye, sirloin, filet mignon, etc.)
- Salt and pepper
- Olive oil
- Optional: garlic, rosemary, or thyme for seasoning

Steps:

1. Preheat your grill to high heat (direct grilling).

2. Season your steak generously with salt and pepper. For extra flavor, rub minced garlic and fresh herbs like rosemary or thyme onto the steak's surface.

3. Lightly brush the steak with olive oil to prevent sticking.

4. Place the steak on the grill grates and cook for a few minutes on each side, turning only once. Use the searing technique mentioned in Chapter 4 to create grill marks and sear the meat.

5. Check the internal temperature with a meat thermometer. For rare, aim for 120°F (49°C); medium-rare, 130°F (54°C); medium, 140°F (60°C); medium-well, 150°F (66°C); well-done, 160°F (71°C).

6. Remove the steak from the grill and let it rest for a few minutes before slicing and serving.

2. Grilled Chicken: Flavorful and Juicy

Grilled chicken is a versatile option, and marinating it can infuse incredible flavors. Here's a simple grilled chicken recipe:

Ingredients:

- Boneless, skinless chicken breasts or thighs
- Marinade (e.g., olive oil, lemon juice, garlic, herbs, and spices)
- Salt and pepper

Steps:

1. Mix the marinade ingredients in a bowl.
2. Place the chicken pieces in a resealable plastic bag or a shallow dish. Pour the

marinade over the chicken, ensuring it's well-coated.

3. Seal the bag or cover the dish and refrigerate for at least 30 minutes, but longer marinating times, even overnight, can yield better results.

4. Preheat your grill to medium-high heat.

5. Remove the chicken from the marinade and season with salt and pepper.

6. Grill the chicken, turning occasionally, until it reaches an internal temperature of 165°F (74°C).

7. Let the chicken rest for a few minutes before serving.

3. Grilled Pork: Tender and Flavorful

Grilled pork offers a wide range of cuts and flavors. Try this simple recipe for grilled pork chops:

Ingredients:

- Pork chops (bone-in or boneless)
- Marinade or dry rub of your choice (e.g., garlic, paprika, brown sugar, soy sauce, and Dijon mustard)
- Salt and pepper

Steps:

1. Prepare the marinade or dry rub according to your preference.
2. Coat the pork chops evenly with the marinade or apply the dry rub generously. Allow the pork chops to marinate for at least 30 minutes.
3. Preheat your grill to medium-high heat.
4. Season the pork chops with salt and pepper.
5. Grill the pork chops for a few minutes on each side until they reach an internal

temperature of 145°F (63°C) for medium-rare.

6. Remove the chops from the grill and let them rest before serving.

4. Grilled Lamb: A Flavorful Delight

Lamb's rich flavor is a perfect match for grilling. Try this recipe for grilled lamb skewers:

Ingredients:

- Lamb cubes (from leg or shoulder)
- Marinade (e.g., olive oil, lemon juice, garlic, oregano, and cumin)

- Salt and pepper
- Wooden skewers (soaked in water)

Steps:

1. Prepare the marinade by mixing the ingredients in a bowl.
2. Thread the lamb cubes onto the soaked wooden skewers.
3. Brush the lamb skewers with the marinade and season with salt and pepper.
4. Preheat your grill to medium-high heat.
5. Grill the lamb skewers, turning occasionally, until they are cooked to your

desired level of doneness. Aim for an internal temperature of 145°F (63°C) for medium-rare.

6. Let the skewers rest briefly before serving.

5. Grilled Sausages: Quick and Flavorful

Sausages are a quick and flavorful option for the grill. Here's how to grill sausages to perfection:

Ingredients:

- Sausages of your choice (e.g., bratwurst, Italian, chorizo, etc.)

Steps:

1. Preheat your grill to medium heat.
2. Place the sausages on the grill grates.
3. Grill the sausages, turning occasionally, until they are browned and cooked through. The internal temperature should reach 160°F (71°C).
4. Remove the sausages from the grill and let them rest for a few minutes before serving.

6. Grilled Kebabs: A Flavor Explosion

Kebabs offer a delightful way to combine meats with vegetables and flavors. Here's a recipe for beef kebabs:

Ingredients:

- Cubed beef (e.g., sirloin or tenderloin)
- Marinade (e.g., soy sauce, Worcestershire sauce, garlic, olive oil, and spices)
- Bell peppers, onions, and cherry tomatoes
- Wooden skewers (soaked in water)

Steps:

1. Prepare the marinade by mixing the ingredients in a bowl.

2. Thread the marinated beef cubes, bell peppers, onions, and cherry tomatoes onto the soaked wooden skewers, alternating between ingredients.

3. Preheat your grill to medium-high heat.

4. Grill the kebabs, turning occasionally, until the beef reaches your desired level of doneness (medium-rare, medium, etc.).

5. Serve the kebabs hot and enjoy the medley of flavors.

7. Grilled Ribs: Falling-off-the-Bone Goodness

Ribs are a barbecue favorite, and grilling them can result in tender, smoky perfection. Try this recipe for grilled ribs:

Ingredients:

- Pork ribs (baby back or spare ribs)
- Dry rub of your choice (e.g., paprika, brown sugar, garlic powder, and cayenne)
- Barbecue sauce (optional)

Steps:

1. Remove the membrane from the back of the ribs for better flavor absorption.

2. Coat the ribs generously with the dry rub, pressing it onto the meat.

3. Preheat your grill to low, indirect heat (around 225°F or 107°C).

4. Place the ribs on the grill grates, bone side down, away from direct heat. Use a smoker box or foil pack with wood chips for added smoky flavor.

5. Close the grill lid and cook the ribs for several hours, maintaining a consistent low

temperature. The ribs are done when they are tender and have pulled back from the bone ends.

6. Optionally, brush the ribs with barbecue sauce in the last 15-30 minutes of cooking for a sticky, sweet glaze.

7. Remove the ribs from the grill, let them rest briefly, and then slice between the bones to serve.

These are just a few examples of the many meat-based grilling recipes you can explore on your grill diet journey. Grilling meats allows you to experiment with a wide range of flavors, seasonings, and cooking techniques to create mouthwatering dishes that will delight your taste buds and impress your family and friends. Whether you're a fan of steak, chicken, pork, lamb, sausages, or ribs, the grill offers endless possibilities for culinary creativity.

CHAPTER 6

Grilling Recipes - Seafood and Vegetables

In Chapter 6 of our exploration into grill diets, we expand our culinary horizons by exploring a variety of grilling recipes beyond meats. Seafood and vegetables take center stage, offering a diverse range of flavors, textures, and health benefits. Grilling seafood and vegetables can be just as satisfying and delicious as grilling meats, if not more so, and this chapter will guide you through some delectable recipes to broaden your grilling repertoire.

1. Grilled Salmon: A Nutrient-Rich Delight

Grilled salmon is a nutritional powerhouse and a crowd-pleaser. Here's a simple recipe for grilled salmon with a lemon-dill marinade:

Ingredients:

- Salmon fillets
- Marinade (e.g., olive oil, lemon juice, garlic, fresh dill, salt, and pepper)

Steps:

1. Prepare the marinade by mixing the ingredients in a bowl.

2. Place the salmon fillets in a resealable plastic bag or shallow dish. Pour the marinade over the salmon and ensure it's well-coated. Refrigerate for at least 30 minutes.

3. Preheat your grill to medium-high heat.

4. Remove the salmon from the marinade and season with additional salt and pepper.

5. Place the salmon fillets on the grill grates, skin side down, and cook for a few

minutes on each side, until the fish flakes easily with a fork.

6. Serve the grilled salmon with fresh lemon wedges for added zest.

2. Grilled Shrimp: Quick and Flavorful

Grilled shrimp are quick to prepare and full of flavor. Try this recipe for garlic-lemon grilled shrimp skewers:

Ingredients:

- Large shrimp, peeled and deveined

- Marinade (e.g., olive oil, lemon zest, minced garlic, fresh parsley, salt, and pepper)

Steps:

1. Mix the marinade ingredients in a bowl.
2. Thread the marinated shrimp onto wooden skewers that have been soaked in water to prevent burning.
3. Preheat your grill to medium-high heat.
4. Grill the shrimp skewers for a few minutes on each side,

until they turn pink and opaque.

5. Serve the grilled shrimp as an appetizer or main dish with additional lemon wedges.

3. Grilled Tuna: A Sushi-Grade Experience

Grilled tuna steaks offer a unique and savory experience. Here's a recipe for grilled tuna with a soy-ginger glaze:

Ingredients:

- Tuna steaks
- Marinade/glaze (e.g., soy sauce, grated ginger, minced

garlic, honey, sesame oil, and red pepper flakes)

- Salt and pepper

Steps:

1. Prepare the marinade/glaze by mixing the ingredients in a bowl.
2. Season the tuna steaks with salt and pepper.
3. Preheat your grill to high heat.
4. Brush the tuna steaks with the marinade/glaze and place them on the grill grates.
5. Grill for just a minute or two on each side, searing the

outside while keeping the interior rare to medium-rare.

6. Serve the grilled tuna steaks with additional glaze drizzled on top.

4. Grilled Vegetables: Healthy and Flavorful

Grilling vegetables can transform them into tender, smoky delights. Here's a basic recipe for grilled mixed vegetables:

Ingredients:

- Assorted vegetables (e.g., bell peppers, zucchini,

eggplant, mushrooms, and red onions)

- Olive oil
- Salt and pepper
- Fresh herbs (e.g., rosemary or thyme) for seasoning

Steps:

1. Preheat your grill to medium-high heat.
2. Cut the vegetables into even-sized pieces for uniform cooking.
3. Toss the vegetables in olive oil, season with salt, pepper, and fresh herbs.
4. Place the vegetables directly on the grill grates or use a

grill basket to prevent them from falling through.

5. Grill the vegetables, turning occasionally, until they are tender and have grill marks.

6. Serve the grilled vegetables as a side dish, in salads, or as a topping for sandwiches and wraps.

5. Grilled Corn: Summer Delight

Grilled corn on the cob is a quintessential summer treat. Here's a recipe for grilled corn with a garlic-herb butter:

Ingredients:

- Fresh corn on the cob, husked
- Butter (softened)
- Minced garlic
- Fresh herbs (e.g., parsley, chives, and basil)
- Salt and pepper

Steps:

1. Preheat your grill to medium-high heat.
2. In a bowl, mix the softened butter, minced garlic, finely chopped fresh herbs, salt, and pepper to create a compound butter.
3. Brush the corn on the cob with the garlic-herb butter.

4. Place the corn directly on the grill grates and cook, turning occasionally, until the kernels are tender and lightly charred.

5. Serve the grilled corn with extra compound butter for spreading.

6. Grilled Portobello Mushrooms: A Vegetarian Delight

Portobello mushrooms are hearty and satisfying when grilled. Try this recipe for balsamic-marinated grilled Portobello mushrooms:

Ingredients:

- Portobello mushroom caps
- Marinade (e.g., balsamic vinegar, olive oil, minced garlic, Dijon mustard, and thyme)
- Salt and pepper

Steps:

1. Remove the stems from the mushroom caps and clean them with a damp paper towel.
2. Mix the marinade ingredients in a bowl.
3. Brush the mushroom caps with the marinade and season with salt and pepper.

4. Preheat your grill to medium-high heat.

5. Grill the Portobello mushrooms for a few minutes on each side until they are tender and have grill marks.

6. Serve the grilled mushrooms as a burger substitute or a side dish.

7. Grilled Asparagus: Simple and Elegant

Grilled asparagus is a simple yet elegant side dish. Here's a recipe for garlic-lemon grilled asparagus:

Ingredients:

- Fresh asparagus spears
- Olive oil
- Minced garlic
- Lemon zest
- Salt and pepper

Steps:

1. Preheat your grill to medium-high heat.
2. Trim the woody ends of the asparagus spears.
3. Toss the asparagus in olive oil, minced garlic, lemon zest, salt, and pepper.
4. Place the asparagus directly on the grill grates or use a grill basket for easy flipping.

5. Grill the asparagus for a few minutes, turning occasionally, until they are tender and have grill marks.

6. Serve the grilled asparagus as a side dish or appetizer.

These seafood and vegetable grilling recipes showcase the versatility and delicious possibilities beyond traditional meat-based grilling. Whether you're a fan of salmon, shrimp, tuna, or a variety of colorful vegetables, the grill allows you to explore a world of flavors and culinary creativity. Incorporating more seafood and vegetables into your grill diet not only adds variety to your meals but also promotes a healthier and more balanced approach to grilling.

CHAPTER 7

Grilling Sauces, Marinades, and Rubs

In Chapter 7 of our exploration into grill diets, we delve into the world of sauces, marinades, and rubs. These flavor-enhancing elements play a crucial role in elevating the taste of your grilled dishes. Whether you're grilling meats, seafood, or vegetables, the right sauce, marinade, or rub can take your culinary creations to the next level. Let's explore the art of creating and using these flavorful additions to your grilling repertoire.

1. Grilling Marinades: Infusing Flavor and Tenderness

Marinades are liquid mixtures that enhance the flavor and tenderness of your grilled items. They typically consist of a few key components:

- **Acid**: Ingredients like vinegar, citrus juice (lemon, lime, orange), or yogurt add acidity, which helps tenderize meat and infuse flavor.

- **Oil**: Olive oil, vegetable oil, or sesame oil are common choices. Oil helps distribute flavors and prevents sticking on the grill.

- **Aromatics**: Garlic, onions, shallots, and fresh herbs add depth and aroma to the marinade.

- **Spices and Herbs**: A combination of spices (like paprika, cumin, and chili powder) and fresh herbs (such as basil, cilantro, or rosemary) provide the desired flavor profile.

- **Sweeteners**: Sugar, honey, or maple syrup can add

sweetness and aid in caramelization.

2. Marinating Tips and Techniques

When using marinades, keep these tips in mind:

- **Marinating Time**: The duration varies depending on the item. Fish and seafood may only need 15-30 minutes, while tougher cuts of meat like beef or lamb can benefit from several hours or even overnight.
- **Container**: Use a resealable plastic bag, shallow dish, or

non-reactive container for marinating. Ensure the food is fully submerged in the marinade.

- **Refrigeration**: Always marinate in the refrigerator, especially for extended periods. Marinating at room temperature can lead to food safety issues.

- **Reserve Marinade**: If you plan to use the marinade for basting or as a sauce, set some aside before adding it to the raw meat or seafood.

3. Grilling Sauces: Adding Flavor and Moisture

Sauces are a fantastic way to add flavor and moisture to grilled items. They can be applied before, during, or after grilling, depending on the recipe. Here are some popular grilling sauces:

- **Barbecue Sauce**: From sweet and smoky to tangy and spicy, barbecue sauce is a classic choice for grilling. It's perfect for brushing onto ribs, chicken, and pork as they cook.

- **Teriyaki Sauce**: Teriyaki sauce combines soy sauce, sake or mirin, sugar, and aromatics. It's great for marinating chicken, beef, or fish.

- **Chimichurri**: This Argentine sauce features fresh parsley, cilantro, garlic, vinegar, and oil. It's excellent for drizzling over grilled steaks or chicken.

- **Salsa**: Salsas come in many varieties, such as mango, pineapple, or tomato. They add a burst of freshness to grilled fish or chicken.

- **Tzatziki**: This Greek sauce made from yogurt, cucumber, garlic, and dill is a perfect complement to grilled lamb or chicken.

4. Applying Sauces While Grilling

When applying sauces during grilling, follow these guidelines:

- **Basting**: Brush the sauce onto your food using a basting brush. Apply it toward the end of the cooking time to prevent burning or caramelization.
- **Glazing**: To create a glossy glaze, apply the sauce in layers, allowing each layer to set before adding more. This technique works well for ribs and chicken wings.

- **Dipping**: Offer sauces as a side or dipping option for your grilled items. This allows guests to control their sauce-to-food ratio.

5. Dry Rubs: Flavorful Coatings

Dry rubs consist of a mixture of dried spices, herbs, and seasonings that are applied directly to the surface of meat or vegetables before grilling. They form a flavorful crust and add dimension to your dishes. Here's how to create and use dry rubs:

- **Ingredients**: Common dry rub ingredients include paprika, chili powder, garlic powder, onion powder, cumin, brown sugar, salt, and pepper.

- **Even Coating**: Ensure an even coating of the dry rub by sprinkling it liberally on all sides of the food and gently pressing it into the surface.

- **Resting Time**: Allow the rubbed meat to rest for at least 15-30 minutes (or longer for more flavor penetration) before grilling.

6. Customizing Your Sauces, Marinades, and Rubs

The beauty of sauces, marinades, and rubs is that they are highly customizable. Here are some ideas for creating your signature flavors:

- **Regional Flavors**: Explore the cuisines of different regions, such as Asian, Mediterranean, Caribbean, or Tex-Mex, to inspire your recipes.

- **Spice Levels**: Adjust the heat level by adding more or less chili powder, pepper, or hot sauce.

- **Sweet and Savory Balance**: Balance sweetness with acidity. For example, pair honey with lemon juice or vinegar.

- **Experiment**: Don't be afraid to experiment with unique ingredients like fruit preserves, whiskey, or specialty vinegars to create unique flavor profiles.

7. Pairing Sauces with Grilled Foods

Consider pairing sauces, marinades, and rubs with specific grilled items to enhance their natural flavors:

- **Steak**: A simple rub of salt, pepper, and garlic works well, but a classic chimichurri sauce adds a burst of freshness.

- **Chicken**: Try marinating chicken in a lemon-herb marinade or glazing it with barbecue sauce.

- **Seafood**: Grilled seafood benefits from a brush of lemon-butter sauce or a drizzle of garlic aioli.

- **Vegetables**: Coat vegetables with olive oil, salt, and pepper before grilling. Serve with a light vinaigrette or herb-infused yogurt sauce.

- **Pork**: For pork, a sweet and smoky barbecue sauce or a Dijon mustard-based marinade can work wonders.

8. Safety and Cross-Contamination

When using sauces, marinades, or rubs, it's essential to practice safe food handling:

- **Cross-Contamination**: Don't reuse marinades that have come into contact with raw meat. If you plan to use the marinade as a sauce, set some aside before marinating the meat.

- **Heat Treatment**: If you've used a marinade on raw meat or seafood, ensure it's brought to a boil before using it as a sauce to kill any potential bacteria.

- **Safe Temperatures**: Always cook meat and seafood to safe internal temperatures, as specified by food safety guidelines.

In this chapter, we've explored the art of creating and using grilling sauces, marinades, and rubs to elevate your grill diet experience.

These flavor-enhancing elements are the secret weapons in your grilling arsenal, allowing you to infuse your grilled dishes with unique tastes and textures. Whether you prefer the bold flavors of barbecue sauce, the subtle nuances of a marinade, or the aromatic richness of a dry rub, mastering the art of sauces and seasonings opens up a world of culinary possibilities on your grill.

CHAPTER 8

Grill Diet - Tips for Success

In Chapter 8, we'll explore essential tips and strategies to ensure your grill diet journey is a resounding success. While grilling is a delightful and healthy way to prepare meals, there are nuances and considerations that can help you get the most out of your grilling experience. Let's dive into these valuable insights to make your grill diet not only delicious but also safe and enjoyable.

1. Grill Safety: A Top Priority

Safety should always come first when grilling. Here are some important safety tips to keep in mind:

- **Location**: Place your grill on a flat, stable surface away from buildings, trees, and overhanging structures. Keep it clear of flammable materials.

- **Check for Gas Leaks**: If you have a gas grill, regularly inspect the hoses and connections for leaks. You can do this by applying a soapy water solution to the connections and watching for bubbles when the gas is on.

- **Ventilation**: Ensure proper ventilation around your grill to prevent the accumulation of carbon monoxide. Grilling in an open area is ideal.

- **Fire Extinguisher**: Have a fire extinguisher nearby, and know how to use it. It's a precaution that can save the day in case of unexpected flare-ups.

- **Supervise the Grill**: Never leave a hot grill unattended. Flames can flare up quickly, and you'll want to be there to manage them.

- **Use Long-Handled Tools**: To avoid getting too close to the heat, use long-handled utensils and tongs when grilling.

2. Preheat the Grill: A Crucial Step

Properly preheating your grill is essential for achieving the right cooking temperature and searing food effectively. Preheating serves several purposes:

- **Cleaning**: It helps burn off any remaining food particles and debris from previous grilling sessions, making it easier to clean the grates.

- **Food Release**: A well-preheated grill prevents food from sticking to the grates, reducing the chances of tearing or losing grill marks.

- **Even Cooking**: It ensures that the entire cooking surface is at the desired temperature, which is critical for even cooking.

3. Use a Meat Thermometer: Precision Matters

Grilling often involves cooking meat to specific internal

temperatures for safety and optimal taste. Using a meat thermometer is the only way to guarantee the right doneness. Here are some general guidelines for safe internal temperatures:

- **Poultry**: Chicken and turkey should reach 165°F (74°C) in the thickest part.
- **Pork**: Pork chops, roasts, and ground pork should reach 145°F (63°C). Ground pork needs special attention, as it can easily harbor bacteria.
- **Beef**: Steaks, roasts, and ground beef should reach a

minimum of 160°F (71°C) for safety. However, many prefer medium-rare steaks, which should be around 130-140°F (54-60°C).

- **Fish**: Fish should reach 145°F (63°C) or until it flakes easily with a fork.
- **Lamb**: Lamb steaks and roasts can be cooked to around 145-160°F (63-71°C) depending on your desired level of doneness.
- **Vegetables**: While vegetables don't require specific internal temperatures for safety, they

should be tender and have nice grill marks.

4. Resting Your Food: Patience Pays Off

After removing meat from the grill, let it rest before cutting or serving. Resting allows the juices to redistribute throughout the meat, resulting in a juicier, more flavorful end product. As a general rule, rest steaks and chops for about 5-10 minutes and larger cuts like roasts for 15-20 minutes.

5. Grilling Vegetables and Fruits: Not Just for Meats

Don't limit your grill to meats alone. Grilling vegetables and fruits can be equally satisfying and healthy. Here are some tips:

- **Preparation**: Brush vegetables and fruits with oil and season with salt and pepper or your choice of herbs and spices.

- **Grill Basket**: For smaller or more delicate items like asparagus or sliced bell peppers, consider using a grill basket to prevent them from falling through the grates.

- **Direct or Indirect Heat**: Depending on the item, you can use both direct and indirect grilling methods. For example, sear vegetables directly over high heat and then move them to a cooler area to finish cooking.

6. Two-Zone Fire: Mastering Temperature Control

A two-zone fire involves creating two distinct temperature zones on your grill:

- **Direct Zone**: One side of the grill is set up for high

heat, ideal for searing and quickly cooking items.

- **Indirect Zone**: The other side of the grill is left without direct heat, providing a cooler area for slow cooking or finishing items that have been seared.

This technique allows for more precise control over cooking and is especially useful when grilling items with varying thicknesses or when you want to keep some food warm while finishing others.

7. Experiment and Adapt: Embrace Creativity

While following recipes and techniques is valuable, don't be afraid to experiment and adapt based on your preferences and available ingredients. Grilling is an art as much as it is a science, and personalization is key to creating memorable dishes.

8. Cleaning and Maintenance: Prolonging Grill Life

Proper grill maintenance ensures longevity and consistent performance. Here are some cleaning and maintenance tips:

- **Clean Grates**: After preheating, use a grill brush

to clean the grates, removing any residue from previous grilling sessions.

- **Empty Ash and Grease Trays**: Regularly empty ash and grease trays to prevent flare-ups and fire hazards.

- **Inspect and Replace Parts**: Check hoses, burners, and other components for wear and tear. Replace them as needed to maintain safety and performance.

- **Cover It**: When not in use, cover your grill to protect it from the elements and extend its lifespan.

- **Deep Clean**: Periodically deep clean your grill by removing the grates and thoroughly cleaning the interior with warm soapy water and a grill brush.

9.   Grilling   for   Health: Balanced Choices

Grilling can be a healthy cooking method, but it's essential to balance your choices. While lean meats, seafood, and grilled vegetables are excellent options, don't overdo processed meats or charred foods, which may carry health risks. Aim for a balanced diet that includes a variety of foods.

10. Share and Enjoy: The Social Aspect of Grilling

Finally, one of the joys of grilling is the social aspect. Whether you're hosting a barbecue with friends or enjoying a family meal, grilling brings people together. Embrace the opportunity to share good food, good company, and good times.

By incorporating these tips and strategies into your grill diet, you'll not only master the art of grilling but also enhance your safety, efficiency, and enjoyment. From perfecting your grilling techniques to experimenting with flavors and ingredients, the grill can become your culinary canvas, allowing you to create delicious and memorable meals for yourself and your loved ones. Happy grilling!

CONCLUSION

In conclusion, our journey through the eight chapters of the "Grill Diet" book has been a flavorful exploration of the world of grilling. From mastering the basics of grilling equipment and techniques to crafting delicious recipes with meats, seafood, vegetables, and flavorful sauces, marinades, and rubs, we've covered the essential elements of a successful grill diet. Along the way, we've also emphasized safety, precision, and creativity to ensure that your grilling experiences are not only delicious but also safe and enjoyable.

Grilling is more than just a cooking method; it's a lifestyle that encourages outdoor gatherings, culinary experimentation, and the enjoyment of fresh, flavorful foods. By following the tips and strategies outlined in this book, you can become a skilled grill master, confidently preparing a wide range of dishes that cater to your tastes and preferences.

Remember that grilling is a versatile and healthy cooking method that allows you to savor the natural flavors of your ingredients while adding a unique smoky touch. It's a way to enjoy a balanced diet that includes lean meats, seafood, and an abundance of vegetables, all while relishing the social aspect of sharing meals with family and friends.

As you embark on your grill diet journey, don't hesitate to adapt and personalize the recipes and techniques to suit your culinary aspirations. Whether you're grilling a perfectly seared steak, a succulent piece of salmon, a colorful medley of vegetables, or experimenting with your own signature marinades and rubs, the grill is your canvas for culinary creativity.

Lastly, cherish the moments spent around the grill, as they often go hand in hand with good company, laughter, and the joy of shared meals. Whether it's a weekend barbecue, a special occasion, or a simple weeknight dinner, grilling can transform ordinary moments into memorable experiences.

With these insights, you're well-equipped to embark on your grill diet adventure, savoring the delicious flavors and the camaraderie that grilling brings. So fire up the grill, gather your loved ones, and let the sizzling and aromatic journey begin. Happy grilling!